Testimonials for
Baby Sleepytime

"After 8 weeks of being up every two hours to comfort my newborn daughter, I was a walking zombie...I tried several different techniques, and the only product that worked for us was *Baby Sleepytime*. The first night I played the disc for my daughter, she slept six consecutive hours. After two weeks of nightly use, she was sleeping nine hours through the night. This disc was a life saver for me...*Baby Sleepytime* is a must-have for every parent!"

> — Amy O. Folkins
> Allen, TX

"I normally have to nurse my baby in order to get him to sleep. [When I used the CD,] he went to sleep in 25 minutes just by holding him."

> — Rachel Dozier
> Dallas,TX

"I had my first child on July 1st, 2007 and...I was very concerned about the baby sleeping through the night. I never imagined that there was a technology product that could so naturally and most effortlessly help baby, mom, and I sleep undisturbed through the entire night. Even when my baby and wife have to wake up to nurse feed, one click of the CD player and we're all quickly right back to sleepy-time again...I would have gladly paid thousands of dollars to bring my family this level of comfort-the value is priceless!"

— James Charles Villepigue

Oyster Bay, NY

"A brilliant gift for parents-to-be and grandparents-to-be! It is fabulous. I get the best night's sleep and feel so rested. I can't say enough good things about *Baby Sleepytime.*"

— Loren Kyle

Dallas, TX

Baby Sleepytime

The CD Scientifically Proven to Put Your Baby to Sleep—Fast

Christopher Oliver

HatherleighPress
New York

HatherleighPress
5-22 46th Avenue, Suite 200
Long Island City, NY 11101
www.hatherleighpress.com

Library of Congress Cataloging-in-Publication Data

Oliver, Christopher.
Baby sleepytime: the CD scientifically proven to put your baby to
sleep—fast / Christopher Oliver.
    p. cm.
 ISBN 978-1-57826-260-1
 1. Infants—Sleep—Popular works. 2. Sleep disorders in
children—Prevention—Popular works. 3. Nursery rhymes. I. Title.
RJ506.S55O45 2007
649'.122--dc22

                         2007023068

Baby Sleepytime is available for bulk purchase, special promotions, and premiums. For information on reselling and special purchase opportunities, call
1-800-528-2550 and ask for the Special Sales Manager.

Interior design by Jasmine Cardoza
Cover design by Kathleen Lynch/Black Cat Design LLC

10 9 8 7 6 5 4 3 2 1
Printed in the United States

Dedication

To my niece, Kaley Emma,
who provided the inspiration behind
Baby Sleepytime.

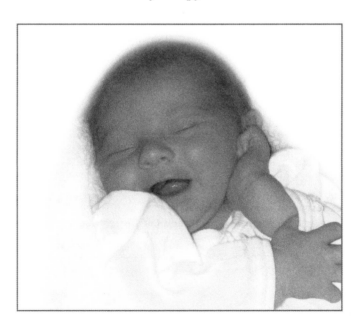

CONTENTS

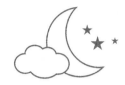

Introduction:
About Baby Sleepytime

As every new parent knows, getting your baby to sleep—and stay asleep—can be much harder than it sounds. My sister's newborn, Kaley Emma, quickly became notorious for waking up frequently. After 8 weeks of being up every two hours, my sister was a walking zombie.

It was about that point, when my sister was frazzled, tired, and just plain worn out, that I came up with the concept behind *Baby Sleepytime*. I had already developed meditation brainwave technologies for adults, so it was a short step from that to create an audio CD with binaural beats to put babies—and adults— right to sleep. The dual binaural beats are mixed with multiple tracks of ocean waves from the Gulf of Mexico, creating a CD that is pleasant to listen to as well as so powerful it will lull your crying baby to dreamland.

And it works! The very first night my sister played the disc for Kaley, she slept for 6 consecutive hours. After just two weeks of nightly use, she was sleeping 9 hours. For a 10-week-old newborn, this seemed miraculous.

I can only imagine how useful this CD can be to you. Just take a minute to pop in the CD, and I guarantee you will be delighted at the results. Never again will you have to spend another night soothing your baby.

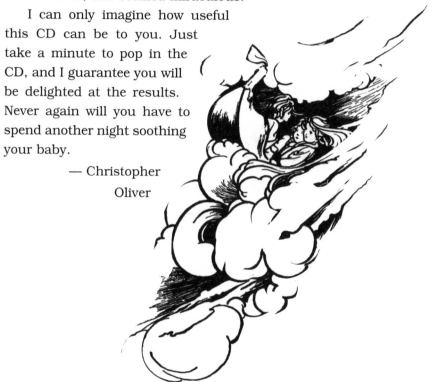

— Christopher
Oliver

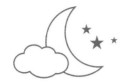

How the CD Technology Works

Employing binaural beat sound technology, this CD is scientifically designed to provide sonic sleep rhythms. Four stereo audio tones blend together, creating six frequencies hidden behind the peaceful sound of ocean waves from the Gulf of Mexico at Padre Island. Designed to work without headphones, it will make your baby—and you—fall asleep faster.

Originally discovered in 1839 by German scientist H. W. Dove, a binaural beat is your brain's way of balancing out two uneven frequencies (such as a 65 Hz pitch to your right ear and an 85 Hz pitch to your left ear). In this example, the binaural beat created by your brain would have the equivalent of 20 Hz, the difference between the two uneven sounds.

These slight mathematical differences between the unique four tones developed for *Baby Sleepytime's* CD are delta frequency range. Your brain automatically translates the dual

binaural tones audio tones into the frequencies encouraging you to relax, rest, rejuvenate, and recharge. This delta frequency is the part of the sleep cycle where deep regenerative sleep takes place, helping you heal and rebuild.

This innovative technique of blending sounds is a direct result of the break-through article in Scientific American in 1973 that introduced binaural beats as inducing the Frequency Following Response (FFR). FFR was first discovered by the scientific world in the 1930s. Research articles on this fascinating subject have also been published in the Journal of Neuroscience (1997), the Journal of Neurophysiology (1998), Physiological Review (2000) and the Handbook of Perception and Cognition (2006).

This proven technology means no more crying and tears at bedtime for babies and no more sleepless nights for you—the parents. Listen with your baby and you'll both be off to dreamland. You'll wake up more relaxed and ener-gized and so will your baby.

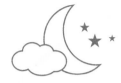

Sleep Tips

The following are a number of soothing techniques that can help your baby quiet down and sleep. (Grandma may know some others).

- **Singing.** A soft lullaby or nursery rhyme. If it works, keep using the same song. Babies enjoy repetition. (See Chapter 4 for some nursery rhymes to read.)
- **Music.** I'm a firm believer in music for people of all ages, including little babies. It's soothing and interesting and makes you feel good. How loud should the music be? If you can't talk over it, it's too loud, which reminds me of a recent wedding we attended.
- **Rhythmic sounds.** The hum of a vacuum cleaner or fan or the rhythm of a dishwasher often calms a baby.
- **Warm bath.** This works for some, but others hate it.

- **Massage.** Again, some babies enjoy being gently stroked, others can't stand it.
- **Cuddling.** This soothing method gives your baby a secure feeling and as far as I'm concerned, the more the better. Kissing while cuddling is highly permissible.
- **Walking the floor.** Carrying your baby around can become tiring, but think of the calories you're burning up.
- **Rhythmic rocking.** In your arms or in an automatic baby swing are effective.
- **Pacifier.** Some babies can only be quieted down with a pacifier. But its important to use a pacifier for the right reason—which means after an adequate feeding when the baby can't settle down and needs some extra sucking. Pacifiers should not be used as a plug to keep the baby quiet.
- **Tummy on lap.** Place your baby on his stomach cross your lap on a heating pad or hot water bottle. At times simply rubbing your babies abdomen helps.
- **Gassiness.** If your baby is crying because of gas, help him expel it with a lubricated rectal thermometer or

infant suppository or by using one of the gas reducing mediations (ask your baby's doctor about them).

- **Automobile ride.** A last resort method, when all else fails. Believe it or not, it works. I will never forget five-month-old Patrick who was driving his parents crazy every day at 1 am. Rain or shine he would start screaming uncontrollably, loud enough to wake up all the neighbors. We tried everything but nothing worked. At 1:30am, I got the phone call and suggested to Patrick's father (home alone with his son) that he go to the all night pharmacy for a mild sedative that I would phone in. You guessed it. They never got to the drugstore. Patrick fell asleep as soon as the care started. There are now devices on the market that simulate the crib going sixty miles an hour that are said to work. I have not had experience with them.

Tips are courtesy of by Alvin N. Eden, M.D., author of *Positive Parenting* (Hatherleigh Press, 2007).

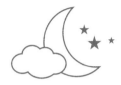

How to Use the Book and CD

Baby Sleepytime has been created to help your baby get to sleep, plus induce longer sleeping periods. *Baby Sleepytime* will easily become an important part of your baby's routine, allowing your infant to quickly achieve deep and restorative sleep.

Read the nursery rhymes as you play the *Baby Sleepytime* CD softly (low volume) on repeat mode in your CD player. While it doesn't matter what size or kind of player you have, it must have stereo speakers for the *Baby Sleepytime* CD to work. Your baby and entire family will enjoy more restful and peaceful nights of deep, healthy sleep.

Nursery Rhymes

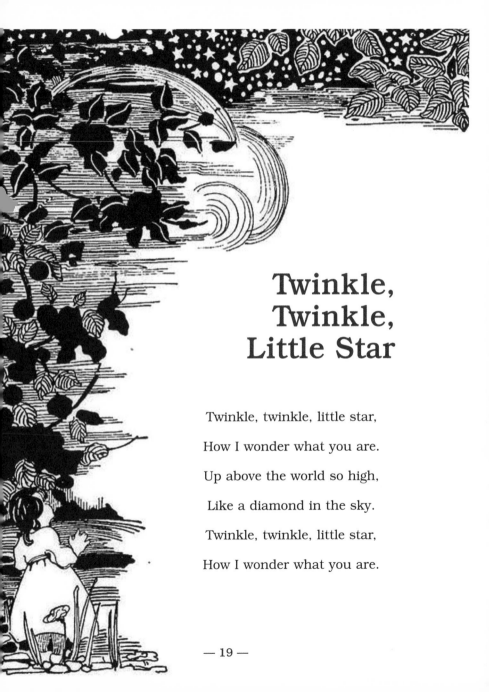

Twinkle, Twinkle, Little Star

Twinkle, twinkle, little star,

How I wonder what you are.

Up above the world so high,

Like a diamond in the sky.

Twinkle, twinkle, little star,

How I wonder what you are.

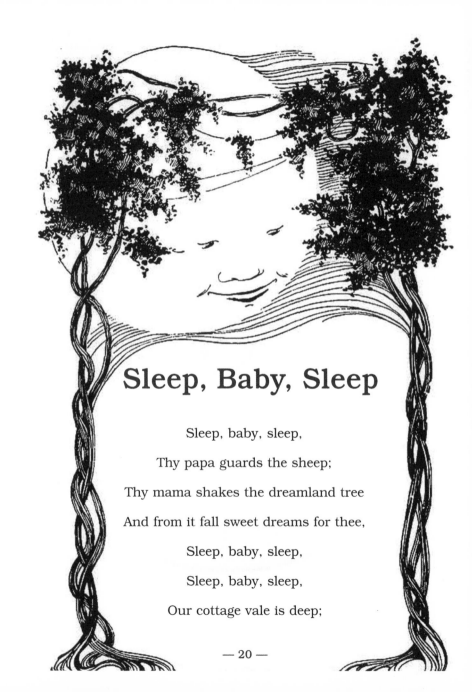

Sleep, Baby, Sleep

Sleep, baby, sleep,

Thy papa guards the sheep;

Thy mama shakes the dreamland tree

And from it fall sweet dreams for thee,

Sleep, baby, sleep,

Sleep, baby, sleep,

Our cottage vale is deep;

The little lamb is on the green,

With woolly fleece so soft and clean,

Sleep, baby, sleep,

Sleep, baby, sleep,

Down where the woodbines creep;

Be always like the lamb so mild,

A kind and sweet and gentle child,

Sleep, baby, sleep.

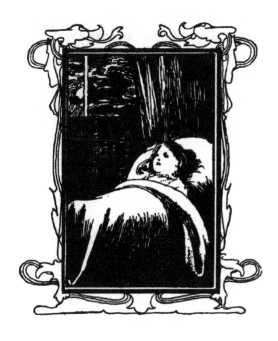

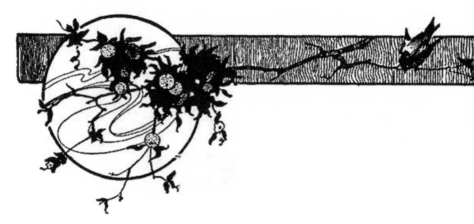

Lullaby, oh, Lullaby

Lullaby, oh, lullaby!

Flowers are closed and lambs are sleeping;

Lullaby, oh, lullaby!

Stars are up, the moon is peeping;

Lullaby, oh, lullaby!

While the birds are silence keeping,

(Lullaby, oh, lullaby!)

Sleep, my baby, fall a-sleeping,

Lullaby, oh, lullaby!

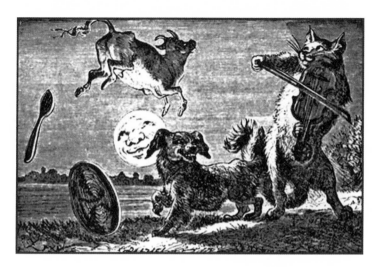

The Man in the Moon

The Man in the moon

Looked out of the moon,

And this is what he said,

'Tis time that, now I'm getting up,

All babies went to bed.

Hey diddle diddle, the cat and the fiddle,

The cow jumped over the moon,

The little dog laughed to see such sport,

And the dish ran away with the spoon.

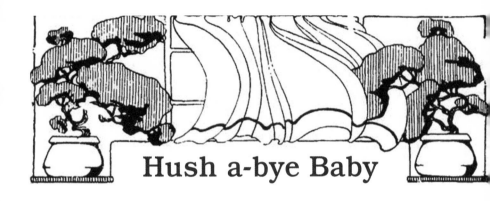

Hush a-bye Baby

Hush-a-bye, baby,

in the tree top.

When the wind blows,

the cradle will rock.

When the bough breaks,

the cradle will fall,

And down will come baby,

cradle and all.

Hush-a-bye, baby,

Your cradle is green,

Daddy's a king,

And Mommy's a queen;

Sister's a lady

Who wears a gold ring;

Brother's a drummer

Who plays for the king.

Hush-a-bye, baby,

Way up on high,

Never mind, baby,

Mommy is nigh,

Swinging the baby

All around—

Hush-a-bye, baby,

Up hill and down.

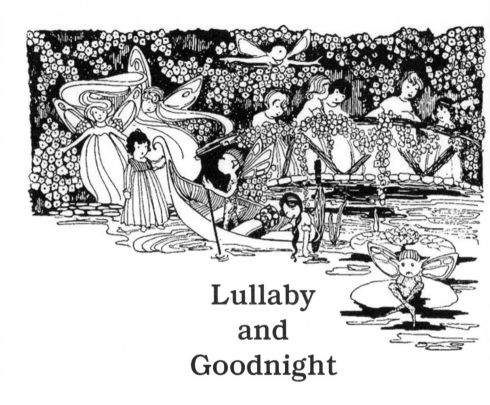

Lullaby
and
Goodnight

Lullaby

And goodnight.

Go to sleep my little baby;

When you wake,

you'll have cake,

and all the pretty little horses.

Black and bays,

Dapples and greys,

Coach and six little horses.

Black and bays,

Dapples and greys,

Coach and six little horses.

Lullaby

And goodnight.

Go to sleep my little baby

Sweet roses, go to sleep

Go to sleep my little baby.

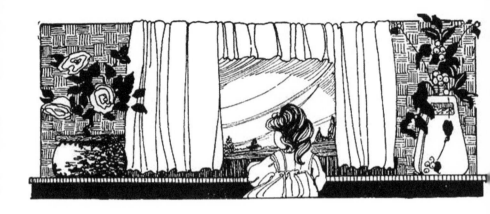

Come to the Window

Come to the window,

My baby, with me,

And look at the stars

That shine on the sea!

There are two little stars

That play bo-peep

With two little fish

Far down in the deep;

And two little frogs

Cry "Neap, neap, neap;"

I see a dear baby

That should be asleep.

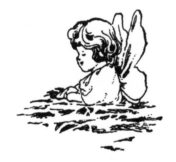

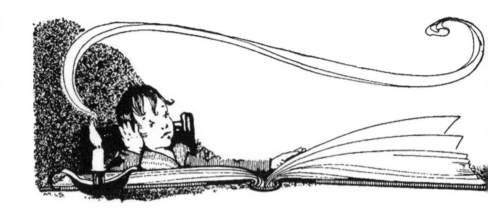

Going to Bed

The evening is coming,

The Sun sinks to rest;

The rooks are all flying

Straight home to their nest.

"Caw!" says the rook, as he flies overhead:

It's time little people were going to bed!

The flowers are closing,

The daisy's asleep;

The primrose is buried

In slumber so deep.

Shut up for the night is the pimpernel red:

It's time little people were going to bed!

The butterfly, drowsy,

Has folded its wing;

The bees are returning,

No more the birds sing.

Their labor is over, their nestlings are fed:

It's time little people were going to bed!

Here comes the pony,

His work is all done;

Down through the meadow

He takes a good run;

Up goes his heels, and down goes his head:

It's time little people were going to bed!

Good-night, little people,

Good-night and good-night;

Sweet dreams to your eyelids,

Till dawning of light;

The evening has come, there's no more to be said:

It's time little people were going to bed!

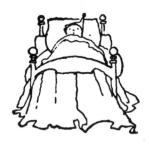

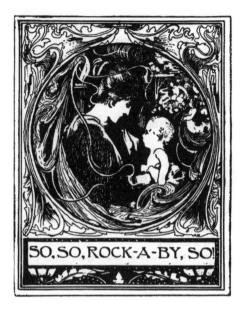

So, So, Rock-a-By So

So, so, rock-a-by so!

Off to the garden where dreamikins grow;

And here is a kiss on your winkiblink eyes,

And here is a kiss on your dimpledown cheek

And here is a kiss for the treasure that lies

In the beautiful garden way up in the skies

Which you seek.

Now mind these three kisses wherever you go-

So, so, rock-a-by so!

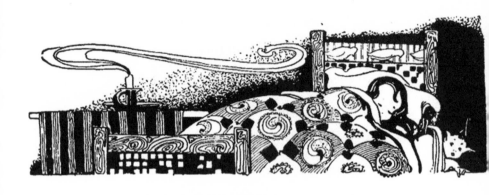

Hush, Little Baby, Don't Say a Word

Hush, little baby, don't say a word,

Papa's gonna buy you a mockingbird

If that mockingbird don't sing,

Papa's gonna buy you a diamond ring

If that diamond ring turns brass,

Papa's gonna buy you a looking glass

If that looking glass gets broke,

Papa's gonna buy you a billy goat

If that billy goat won't pull,

Papa's gonna buy you a cart and bull

If that cart and bull turn over,

Papa's gonna buy you a dog named Rover

If that dog named Rover won't bark,

Papa's gonna buy you a horse and cart

If that horse and cart fall down,

You'll still be the sweetest little baby in town.

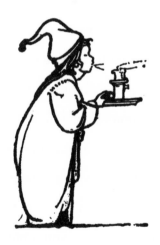

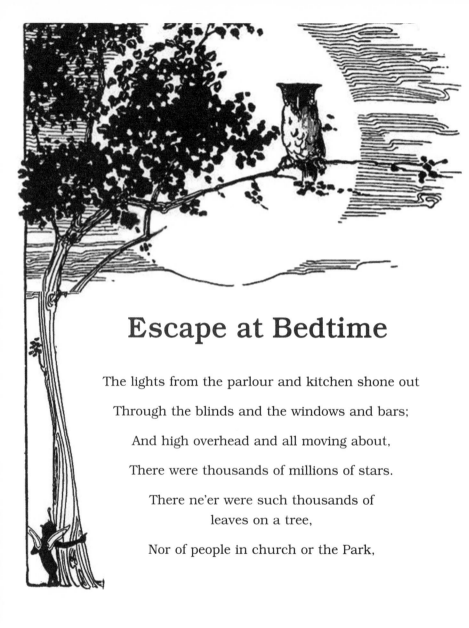

Escape at Bedtime

The lights from the parlour and kitchen shone out

Through the blinds and the windows and bars;

And high overhead and all moving about,

There were thousands of millions of stars.

There ne'er were such thousands of
leaves on a tree,

Nor of people in church or the Park,

As the crowds of the stars that looked
down upon me,

And that glittered and winked in the dark.

The Dog, and the Plough, and the Hunter, and all,

And the star of the sailor, and Mars,

These shown in the sky, and the pail by the wall

Would be half full of water and stars.

They saw me at last, and they chased me with cries,

And they soon had me packed into bed;

But the glory kept shining and bright in my eyes,

And the stars going round in my head.

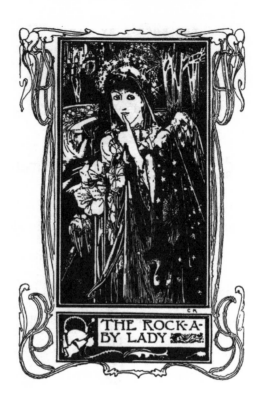

THE ROCK-A-BY LADY

The Rock-a-By Lady

The Rock-a-By Lady from Hushaby Street

Comes stealing, comes creeping;

The poppies they hang from her head to her feet

And each hath a dream that is tiny and fleet,

She brings her poppies to you, my sweet,

When she finds you sleeping!

There is one little dream of a beautiful drum,

"rub-a-dub!" it goes:

There is one little dream of a big sugar-plum,

And lo, thick and fast the other dreams come,

Of pop guns that bang, and tin tops that hum,

And a trumpet that blows.

And dollies peep out of those wee little dreams

With laughter and singing;

And boats go a-floating on silvery streams,

And the stars peek-a-boo with their own misty gleams,

And up, up and up, where the Mother Moon beams,

The fairies go winging!

Would you dream all these dreams that are tiny and fleet?

They'll come to you sleeping;

So shut the two eyes that are weary, my sweet,

For the Rock-a-by Lady from Hushaby Street,

With poppies that hang from her head to her feet,

Comes stealing, comes creeping.

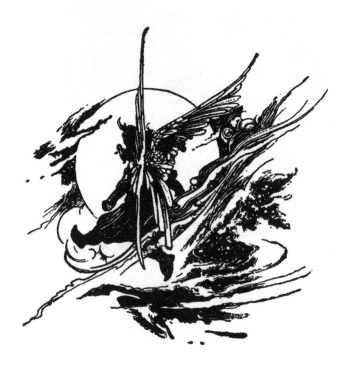

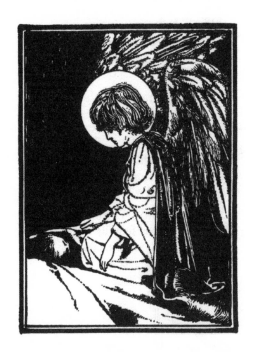

Fairy and Child

Oh, listen, little Dear-My-Soul,

To the fairy voices calling,

For the moon is high in the misty sky

And the honey dew is falling;

To the midnight feast in the clover bloom

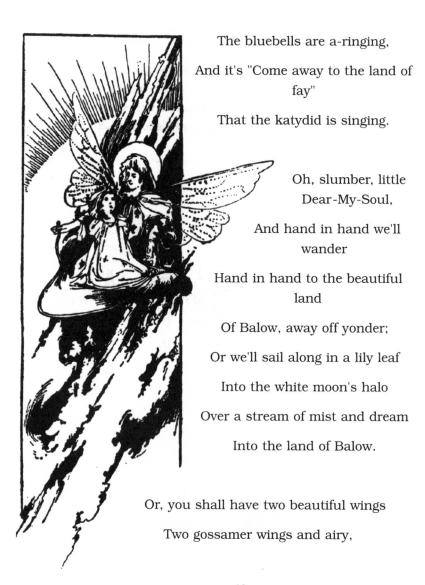

The bluebells are a-ringing,

And it's "Come away to the land of fay"

That the katydid is singing.

Oh, slumber, little Dear-My-Soul,

And hand in hand we'll wander

Hand in hand to the beautiful land

Of Balow, away off yonder;

Or we'll sail along in a lily leaf

Into the white moon's halo

Over a stream of mist and dream

Into the land of Balow.

Or, you shall have two beautiful wings

Two gossamer wings and airy,

And all the while shall the old moon smile

And think you a little fairy;

And you shall dance in the velvet sky,

And the silvery stars shall twinkle

And dream sweet dreams as over their beams

Your footfalls softly tinkle.

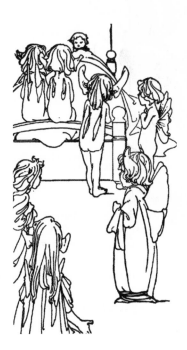

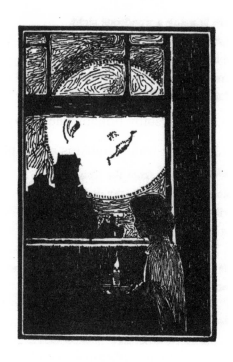

Orkney Lullaby

A moonbeam floateth from the skies,

Whispering, "Heigho, my dearie!

I would spin a web before your eyes-

A beautiful web of silver light,

Wherein is many a wondrous sight

Of a radiant garden leagues away,

Where the softly tinkling lilies sway,

And the snow-white lambkins are at play-

Heigho, my dearie!"

A brownie stealeth from the vine

Singing, "Heigho, my dearie!

And will you hear this song of mine-

A song of the land of murk and mist

Where bideth the bud the dew hath kist?

Then let the moonbeam's web of light

Be spun before thee silvery white,

And I shall sing the livelong night-

Heigho, my dearie!"

The night wind speedeth from the sea,

Murmuring, "Heigho, my dearie!

I bring a mariner's prayer for thee;

So let the moonbeam veil thine eyes,

And the brownie sing thee lullabies;

But I shall rock thee to and fro,

Kissing the brow he loveth so,

And the prayer shall guard thy bed, I trow-

Heigho, my dearie!"

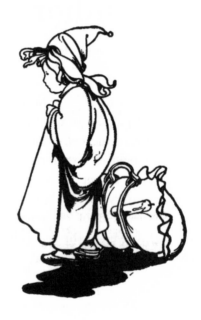

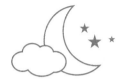

About the Author

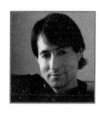

Christopher Oliver is America's foremost developer and pioneer of cutting-edge motivational, relaxation, and meditation products. He is the creator of the extraordinary *AV3X: Digital Meditation* series (www.av3x.com) and other revolutionary brainwave entrainment technologies. A guru in the field of consciousness technology, Christopher has been involved in the mind/body health industry since the early 1990s.